THE COMPLETE
#2020
LOW CARB
COOKBOOK

Lose Weight with Quick and Healthy Recipes for Every Day incl. Delicious Low Carb Desserts

Charlotte M. Gardner

ISBN - 9798617576667

INTRODUCTION

What is Low Carb?

A low carb diet is basically a diet consisting of foods low in carbohydrates which are primarily found in food items such as bread, pasta and sugary foods in general. A low carb diet essentially replaces these foods with healthier alternatives and whole foods rich in natural protein, vegetables, and fat. It has been shown from several studies that a low carbohydrate diet can help in achieving weight loss goals and improving one's health markers as well. A low carb diet has been recommended for years for various people by physicians and dietitians. They are simple and easy to follow with no need to count calories or buy any special products.

Is Low Carb really healthy?

A low carb diet requires you to eat fewer carbohydrates and more fats and protein. While many people have been led to think that fat is detrimental to health, new studies have revealed this is not entirely true. In fact, a low-fat diet typically consists of food that is full of sugar which is unhealthy and can lead to health problems like obesity, diabetes complications and so on. In essence, it is safe to conclude that natural fat is not the enemy. Instead, living on a low carb diet is a healthier alternative.

A low carb diet helps you to cut down on starches and sugar. This helps to stabilize your blood sugar level and reduce the level of insulin which acts as a fat-storing hormone. A low diet is also essential for weight loss. By consuming fewer carbohydrates, your body will turn to its excess fat reserve as a source of energy thus inducing weight loss naturally and healthily. Low carb foods are also more filling as you feel a lot more satiated while eating less. This reduces food intake and helps to achieve healthy weight loss faster.

However, althouh a low carb diet is healthy for a lot of people doesn't mean it is safe for everyone. You should not go on a strict low-carb diet if you are taking medication for diabetes or high blood pressure. A low carbohydrate diet is also not recommended for nursing/breastfeeding mothers.

What am I allowed to eat?

A low carb diet limits the proportion of carbohydrates in your meals. Instead, you are allowed to eat food rich in proteins, healthy fats, fruits, and vegetables. Below are some of foods you are free to eat on a low-carbohydrate diet.

Meat: Any type of meat is allowed. These include beef, pork, lamb, poultry, game meat and so on. You are also allowed to eat the fats on the meats as well. However, grass-fed meats or organics are more recommended.

Fish and seafood: a low carb diet permits all kinds of fish and seafood. As an additional benefit, fatty fish like mackerel, salmon, herrings, and sardines are rich in omega-3 which is highly recommended.

Vegetables: on a low carbohydrate diet, you are allowed to eat all types of vegetables that grow above the ground. This includes broccoli, cauliflower, kale, Brussels sprouts, spinach, zucchini, eggplant, spinach, mushrooms, olives, onions, avocado, lettuce, tomatoes, and so on. They contain low net carbs and can be freely incorporated into your meals.

Fruits: there are restrictions on the types of fruits you can take on a low carb diet. This is because most fruits are rich in carbs a huge portion of which comes from fibers. For example, an apple contains as much as 21 grams of carbs and so should not be included in your low-carb routine. However, nuts and berries are great and can be included as treats.

Eggs and dairy products: you can include egg in your carb diet whether as boiled, fried, scrambled or as omelets. Feel free to include full-fat dairy products as well as cream, butter, yogurt and cheeses. They help to keep you satiated and full. However, you may want to avoid or limit your intake of regular milk, skim milk and reduced-fat milk as they contain lots of sugar.

What to keep one's hands-off

A low carb diet as the name implies means you limit the proportion of carbohydrates in your meals. This means food that is particularly high in carbohydrates and sugars should be avoided entirely or limited. Some of the common foods you should keep your hands off include:

Bread: avoid or limit both whole grain or refined flour bread. White bread, whole-wheat bread, bagels, and others should be removed from your diet entirely or taken only once in a while as a single sandwich or burrito will easily take you near your daily carb limit.

Grains: most grainy foods should be avoided as well. Rice, oats, wheat and other grains contain high amounts of carbohydrates and should be limited.

Fruits: as earlier mentioned, fruits are high in sugar and fiber. Thus they should not be included in your low-carb meals at all. If you will eat fruits at all, nut and berries are the recommended option since they are generally considered low carb.

Starchy vegetables: keep your hands off certain types of vegetables that are rich in starch as they contain more carbohydrates than fiber. These include potatoes, corn. Beets and so on.

Pasta: 1 cup of cooked pasta may contain as much as 43 grams of carbohydrates. Hence, you should avoid pasta entirely or limit consumption to very small portions.

Other types of foods you should avoid on a low carb diet include cereals, sweetened yogurt, and other dairy products, juice and beer, beans and other legumes, sugar in any form at all, crackers and chips and so on. You can easily find alternatives to these food items or limit consumption to the barest minimum if they cannot be avoided entirely.

How many Carbs per Day?

There is, in fact, no strict definition of how much carbohydrates constitute a low carb diet. However, generally, you should keep your daily carbohydrate intake to a maximum of 100 to 150grams. However, for optimum results, you should target a range of 20 to 50grams daily.

How to start with Low Carb?

A low carb diet is easy and convenient to begin. You don't even need to know how to track or calculate calories. All that is required is a basic knowledge of the low carb ingredients you are permitted to include in your meals and the high carb ones you are expected to avoid. Here are some simple tips that will help you get started.

Know the low carb ingredients to eat and the ones to avoid: the first step to get started whether you are cooking your own meals or not is to know the low carb foods and the high-carb ones you want to avoid. This will guide you in knowing what to include in your meals and the healthier alternatives to the high carb foods that you want to avoid.

Know how to track the carb counts for various servings sizes of food: the goal here is to ensure that you are getting a low carb count while still enjoying optimal nutritional value on the food you are being served. Hence, you should get familiar with how much carb is contained in a plate of food you eat. Not that foods with the same carbohydrate count may not be equal in terms of nutritional value. hence, you should still go food that will supply ample protein and other important nutrients you will be needing despite the low carbohydrate content.

Prepare a meal plan: creating a meal plan ahead will help you organize your meals. You can set up a daily or weekly meal plan that will make it easier to decide on what to eat. Your meal plan will guide your trip to the grocery store and what you cook for each meal. Planning your meals in advance this way is important if you want to stick to a diet and avoid unhealthy food choices. Similarly, you can also prepare your meals ahead of time using meal preps that can be easily kept frozen for future meals.

Meal preps make cooking more convenient and make it easier to follow your diet even when your schedule gets busy.

Take low carb snacks with you: your low carb diet isn't restricted to your main meals, there are low carb snacks as well and you should carry them along with you and take them in between meals. Eating low carb snacks will also help you regulate how much you eat during your main meals and prevents overeating.

Try carb cycling: this method involves eating food with very low carbohydrate content for some days followed by a day of eating higher carb meals. This is a smart way to keep your body healthy as it reduces the chances of your body going into fat-burning plateaus due to a low carb diet.

Know the different forms of carbs: there are various forms of carbohydrates and you should get familiar with them. Simple carbs such as white flour and white sugar contain sugars that are easy to digest. Processed carbs, on the other hand, are harder to process and are not recommended for people who are just starting out on a low carb diet. Even when taking simple carbs, you should recognize the fact that the nutritional composition of these foods may vary from one to the other. You should target low carb foods that are still loaded with essential nutrients needed for health and proper body functioning.

Know the alternatives: knowing how to substitute high-carb ingredients for low carb ones is an important skill to successfully follow your low carb diet. For example, instead of taco shells, you can use lettuce leaves or use spaghetti squash in place of noodles. Zucchini ribbons can also substitute for pasta and you can use cauliflower for pizza crust. Learning how to substitute ingredients this way is important to make it easier to follow a low-carb diet and still enjoy some of the meals you love.

Be aware of risks: while a low carb diet offers several benefits, there are major limitations you should note. For example, while exercise is good for overall health, people on a low carb diet are usually advised to avoid intense activities. Intense activities. Such rigorous exercises or activities require extra endurance and a lot of carbohydrates to serve as fuel. Hence you should limit these activities or avoid them entirely if you intend to start a low carb diet. Other potential risks of a low carb diet include nausea, cramping, constipation, high cholesterol, palpitations, weakness, headaches and so on. It may also lead to some long term health issues like nutritional deficiency, reduced bone density, gastrointestinal issues and so on.

A low carb diet offers several benefits. However, a lot of planning is involved if you will get optimal results. If you intend to begin a low-carb diet you should see a doctor and confirm if you are not at any risk of complications. You can also see a nutritionist for tips on how to transition to a low carb diet healthily.

RECIPES

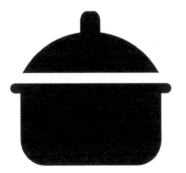

BREAKFAST RECIPES

LOW-CARB BREAD

TIME: 45 MINUTES
AMOUNT: 12 SERVINGS

Calories-294
Protein-14g
Fat-24g
Carbs-6g

INGREDIENTS:

- Yolk and egg white (from 6 eggs)
- Almond flour (2c)
- Whole eggs (2)
- Oil (1/3c)
- Baking powder (1 tbsp)
- Cream of tartar (1/4 tsp)
- Salt (added to taste)

How to prepare

| 1 | Get oven ready by preheating to 375F/190C |

| 2 | Separate 6 egg yolks and whites and place them in two separate medium sized bowls. |

| 3 | Break and pour the 2 eggs into a bowl with the yolks then add oil. Beat or whisk mixture till smooth. |

| 4 | To this, add baking powder, almond flour and salt. Stir mixture till well combined and set aside. |

| 5 | To the bowl of egg whites, add cream of tarter and beat using a hand mixture until it forms stiff peaks. |

| 6 | Transfer 1/3 of the whipped egg-cream mixture to the almond flour batter using a rubber spatula then fold in. Repeat this for the next 1/3 of the egg whites and fold in again. |

7   Add the last batch of 1/3 of egg whites and fold in until smooth.

8   Prepare a loaf pan by lining the bottom with parchment sheet then pour in batter

9   Bake bread for 40 minutes till a golden crust is formed.

10 Turn oven off and set bread aside to cool for about 10 minutes. Remove bread from pan with a thin knife

11 Set aside to cool for a while before you slice and serve.

CAULIFLOWER-CRUSTED QUICHE

TIME: 1 HOUR 20 MINS
AMOUNT: 8 SERVINGS

Calories-219kcal
Protein-16g
Fat-12g
Carbs-11g

INGREDIENTS:

- Parmesan (1/2c)
- Cauliflower (1 head, cut into florets)
- Salt (3/4 tsp)
- Eggs (6 divided)
- Milk (1 cup)
- Garlic powder (1/4 tsp)
- Feta cheese (1/2 cup)
- Olive oil (1/2 tsp)
- Asparagus (8 spears)
- Pepper (1/2 tsp)
- Baby spinach (4c)
- Chopped green onions (3)

HOW TO PREPARE:

12 Get oven ready by preheating to 400F/225C

13 Add cauliflower into a food processor/blender then blitz to form fine crumbs. Pour cauliflower crumbs into a microwave-safe dish. Place dish in microwave for 5 minutes. remove then leave to cool.

14 Place cauliflower into a towel and squeeze out as much water from it as you can.

15 Pour cauliflower into a medium bowl. Add egg, cheese and garlic powder into the bowl then season with 1/4 tsp salt.

16 Press the crust into a tart plate. Ensure that it goes up on the sides of the tart plate.

17 Place in oven and bake for about 15 to 18 minutes till it turns a golden color then leave aside to cool.

18 Turn oven temperature down to 375°F (190°C).

19 Mix 5 eggs, feta cheese, pepper & salt in a different bowl.

20 In a medium skillet, heat oil. Cook asparagus in the oil for a few minutes to tenderize. Add the spinach then cook until wilted.

21 Place the spinach and asparagus mixture at the base of the cooked cauliflower crust. Over this, pour the egg & cheese mixture and sprinkle with onions

22 Put in the oven and leave to bake for 40 to 45 minutes until quiche tuns a slight golden color. Leave for about 15 minutes to cool then serve.

BAKED AVOCADO EGGS

TIME: 30 MINS
AMOUNT: 4 SERVINGS

Calories-271kcal
Protein-12g
Fat-21g
Carbs-7g

INGREDIENTS:

- ◆ Avocados (2)
- ◆ Eggs (4)
- ◆ Bacon bits (1/4c)
- ◆ Cherry tomato (1, quartered)
- ◆ Salt & pepper (to taste)
- ◆ Fresh basil (1 sprig, chopped)
- ◆ Fresh chives (chopped, 2 tbsp)

HOW TO PREPARE

| 1 | Preheat the oven to 200C/380F |

| 2 | Slice avocados into halves and remove the pit of each |

| 3 | Place the avocado halves on a parchment sheet. Scoop out some flesh to create a bigger hole |

| 4 | Crack one egg into each hole. Add a pinch of salt and pepper to taste then add tomato, bacon bits and other toppings as desired |

| 5 | Put in an oven then leave to bake for 13 to 15 minutes till the yolk is at a desired consistency. |

| 6 | Sprinkle fresh herbs as desired. |

SAUSAGE & EGG BREAKFAST CUPS

TIME: 45MINUTES
AMOUNT:4 SERVINGS

Calories-502kcal
Protein-33g
Fat-39g
Carbs-2g

INGREDIENTS:

- Ground sausage (1lb or 0.45kg, chicken, pork, or turkey)
- Onion powder (1/4 tsp)
- Salt and pepper (as desired)
- Garlic powder (1/4 tsp)
- Parsley (1/4 tsp, dried)
- Eggs (6)
- Paprika (1/4 tsp)
- For filling:
- Cheddar cheese (added to taste)
- Tomato (diced)
- Spinach (chopped)

HOW TO COOK:

1   Mix all the ingredients (apart from the egg, pepper and salt) in a bowl then whisk till fully combined.

2   Prepare muffin tins and fill them with the sausage mix. Ensure that the sides are covered by leave some space in the middle where the egg mixture will be added later..

3   In another bowl, mix egg, pepper and salt.

4   Pour egg mixture in the space left earlier at the center of each muffin cup.

5   Add tomatoes, spinach and cheddar cheese with any other toppings of your choice.

6   Place the muffin tins in an oven the bake for 24-30 minutes.

7   Remove from the oven then serve.

HAM & CHEDDAR WRAPPED BREAKFAST BURRITO

TIME: 30 MINUTES
AMOUNT: 1 SERVING

Calories-502kcal
Protein-33g
Fat-39g
Carbs-2g

INGREDIENTS:

♦ Eggs (2)

♦ Salt (as desired)

♦ Parmesan (1 tbsp)

♦ Cheddar cheese (1/4c,shredded)

♦ Butter (1/2 tbsp)

♦ Ham (3 slices)

♦ Scallion (2 tbsp, sliced)

HOW TO PREPARE:

1	Whisk eggs and Parmesan cheese inside a bowl until well mixed. Add salt to taste.
2	Melt butter in a saucepan over medium heat. Pour in the egg mixture.
3	Leave the egg to cook till it starts to set.
4	Add in ham, cheddar cheese and scallion into the center of the egg wrap
5	Cook for about 4 minutes with the lid covered till the egg is well cooked and cheese has melted.
6	Remove form the pan then fold egg wrap beginning with the left and right sides. Roll from the bottom to top to form burrito.
7	Serve and enjoy.

QUICK LOW CARB FRENCH TOAST

TIME: 10 MINUTES
AMOUNT: 1 SERVING

Calories-344kcal
Protein-11g
Fat-28g
Carbs-11g

INGREDIENTS:

- 1 egg
- Butter (1 tbsp)
- Almond milk(3 tbs unsweetened)
- Almond flour (3 tbsp)
- Vanilla extract (1 tsp)
- Baking powder (1/4 tsp)
- Cinnamon (or maple syrup or any sugar free sweetener)

HOW TO COOK:

1 To prepare batter, melt butter and leave to cool in a jug.

2 Whisk egg and add into batter. Add the almond milk & vanilla extract. Also add in baking powder, coconut flour and almond flour. The bread formed should be spongy and soft with no liquid.

3 Turn bread onto a counter top or chopping board. Slice half horizontally into two slices.

4 Melt butter in a skillet. Fry bread in oil over medium high heat for 3 minutes on each side.

5 Serve with topping as desired.

LOW CARB BREAKFAST CASSEROLE

TIME: 45 MINUTES
AMOUNT: 9 SERVINGS

Calories-281kcal
Protein-17g
Fat-23g
Carbs-1g

INGREDIENTS:

- Breakfast sausage (1lb/0.45kg)
- Minced Garlic (6 cloves)
- Cheddar cheese (2 cups, divided)
- Eggs (12)
- Sea salt (1/4 tsp)
- Heavy cream (1/2c)
- Fresh parsley (2 tbsp, chopped)
- Broccoli-optional (3 cups, cut into florets)
- Black pepper (1/4 tsp)

HOW TO COOK:

1   Grease a skillet and set over medium high heat. Cook minced garlic in skillet until fragrant.

2   Add breakfast sausage then cook for 7 to 10 minutes till browned. Use a spatula to break apart as you cook.

3   Heat oven to 375F/190C

4   Blanch broccoli or any other veggies with boiling water for about 5 to 8 minutes till tender and crisp then plunge into ice bath. Drain broccoli then pat dry.

5   Mix eggs, parsley, half of cheddar cheese, heavy cream, salt and black pepper in a bowl.

6   Grease the base of a glass or ceramic cassarole dish. Arrange crumbled sausage at the bottom of this dish evenly. Mix in cooked vegetables with the sausage.

7   Pour in egg mixture over sausage then add the remaining 1/2 of the cheddar cheese.

8   Bake in oven for 25 to 30 minutes till eggs are set and the cheese melts.

LOW CARB ALMOND AND BLUEBERRY SHAKE

TIME: 5 MINUTES
AMOUNT: 1 SERVING

Calories-149kcal
Protein-4g
Fat-11g
Carbs-9g

INGREDIENTS:

♦ Unsweetened almond milk (1 cup)

♦ Fresh blueberries (1/4 cup)

♦ Creamy almond butter (unsweetened, 1 cup)

♦ Maple syrup

HOW TO MAKE:

1 Pour all your ingredients into a jar then blend with a stick blender until smooth

2 Taste for sweetness. You can add syrup if desired

3 Pour smoothie into a glass & serve.

MEXICAN BREAKFAST CASSEROLE

TIME: 40 MINUTES
AMOUNT: 8 SERVINGS

Calories-515kcal
Protein-31g
Fat-42g
Carbs-4g

INGREDIENTS:

- Whole eggs (12)
- Poblano peppers (1/2 cup roasted & chopped)
- Onions (minced, 1/4 cup)
- Shredded cheddar cheese (2 cups)
- Tomatoes (1/3 cup)
- Garlic salt (1 tsp)
- Heavy cream (1/3 cup)
- Cilantro2 tbsp plus more for garnish, freshly chopped)
- Cayenne pepper (1/2 tsp)
- Queso fresco & fresh avocado slices for toppings.

HOW TO COOK:

1 Switch oven to broil. Place poblano peppers in a sheet pan that has been lined with baking sheet and oil lightly. Roast in oven till the skin become charred.

2 Remove from oven then set aside in a glass bowl. Cover with a plastic wrap. This will make it easier to peel off the skin later.

3 After a few minutes, peel the skin off the peppers, remove seeds then chop.

27

4 Turn down temperature of the oven to 180C/350F

5 Cook chorizo sausage in a skillet till browned. While chorizo is being browned, mix eggs using a hand whisk or immersion blender.

6 Drain chorizo and remove from heat and add it to the bowl containing the eggs.

7 Saute onions fora while then add in egg mixture along with the remaining ingredients (keep 1 cup of the cheddar cheese aside)

8 Pour them mixture into a casserole baking dish prepared by spraying with non-stick oil.

9 Add remaining shredded cheddar cheese as topping. Bake in the oven for 30 to 35 minutes till eggs set.

10 Leave to cool slightly before cutting and serving with toppings.

ALMOND FLOUR PANCAKES (LOW-CARB)

TIME: 30 MINUTES
AMOUNT: 5 SERVINGS

Calories-302kcal
Protein-15g
Fat-25g
Carbs-8g

INGREDIENTS:

- Almond flour (1 cup)
- Erythritol (1/4 cup)
- Bakingpowder (3/4 tsp)
- Coconut flour (1/4 cup)
- Whey protein (3 tbsp)
- Salt (1/2 tsp)
- Coconut milk (7 oz/200g, full fat)
- Coconut oil (2 tbsp)
- Egg white (from1 egg)
- Stevia glycerite (1/4 tsp)
- Eggs (2)
- Vanilla extract (1/2 tsp)

HOW TO COOK:

1   Measure all the dry ingredient into a bowl and blend using a hand mixer.

2   Add the wet ingredients into the bowl of blended dry ingredients & mix with a hand mixer.

3   Place a skillet over medium high heat. Spray skillet & pour in pancake.

4   batter with a small ladle or measuring cup.

5 Spread batter evenly to form a circular pancake that is about 3 to 4 inches across.

6 Cook pancake until a skim is forms around its edges, flip then cook.

7 Serve when it is done.

LUNCH RECIPES

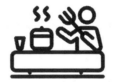

CLOUD BREAD

TIME: 35 MINUTES
AMOUNT:8 SERVINGS

Calories-59kcal
Protein-5g
Fat-11g
Carbs-0.2g

INGREDIENTS:

- Butter or oil (for greasing)
- Eggs (4, separated)
- Cream cheese (1/4 tsp)
- Cream of tarter (1/4 tsp)
- Nigella seeds(1/2 tsp)
- Pepper & salt -as desired

HOW TO MAKE:

1 Preheat your oven to 150C/350F and get baking sheets ready by greasing with oil or butter

2 Whisk egg whites in bowl using an electric beater until stiff peaks begin to form. (you should be able to turn the bowl upside down carefully without its content falling out)

3 In different bowl, mix egg bowl, cream of tarter and the cream cheese using a beater till the mixture becomes frothy and smooth.

4 Fold egg whites one spoonful at a time into the yolk mixture. Do this as gently as possible so that you do not knock out too much air as you do so.

5 Fold in the nigella seeds and add pepper & salt to taste

6 Carefully dollop the mixture on baking sheet. (leave the last few spoonfuls in the bowl because they may be runny)

7   Place in oven and bake bake for 17 to 20 minutes till the bread is craggy at the top and turns a light golden color.

8   Turn oven off and leave to cool before carefully removing the bread from the paper using a palette knife.

9   Cloud bread can be served as a low-carb option for sandwiches.

PAILLARD OF CHICKEN WITH LEMON & HERBS

TIME: 20 MINUTES
AMOUNT: 6 SERVINGS

Calories-240kcal
Protein-32g
Fat-13g
Carbs-1g

INGREDIENTS:

- Olive oil (2 tbsp)
- Chicken breasts (skinless)
- Bag rocket (140g/6oz)
- Balsamic vinegar (1/2 tsp)
- Parmesan (35g/1oz)
- Lemon wedges
- Garlic (2 cloves)
- Rosemary sprigs (2, chopped finely)
- Sage leaves (6, finely chopped)
- Lemon zest (1 lemon)
- Olive oil (3 tbsp)
- Juice (from 1/2 lemon)

HOW TO COOK:

1 Place each piece of chicken breasts between 2 baking sheets or cling film. Bash each piece with a rolling pin or mallet until flattened out with an even layer that is about 0.5cm thick. Transfer mashed meat to a bowl.

2 Prepare marinade by crushing garlic and add salt to taste. Add sage and rosemary and crush together by pounding. Add lemon zest, juice, olive oil and some ground pepper. Pour the marinade over chicken until well coated. Cover & leave for about 2 hours to chill. (you can prepare for 2 hours prior to cooking)

3   Heat barbecue and spread coal to an even layer after the flames have died down. Cook chicken for 3 minutes on both sides. Transfer cooked meat to a board and leave to rest.

4   Mix oil and balsamic vinegar in a bowl. Add rocket and season. Toss together then shave over Parmesan cheese. This can be served as salad with the liquid along with some lemon wedges.

PRAWN AND CRAB COCKTAIL LETTUCE CUPS

TIME: 30 MINUTES
AMOUNT: 8 SERVINGS

Calories-162kcal
Protein-12g
Fat-10g
Carbs-5g

INGREDIENTS:

For Marie rose sauce

- Mayonnaise (4 tbsp)
- Tomato ketchup (3 tbsp)
- Worcestershire sauce (2 tsp)
- Juice and zest (from 1 lemon)
- Cayenne (a pinch)

For tomato salsa

- Tomatoes (4, seeds removed and diced)
- Red onion (1, finely diced)
- Tobasco (1 1/2 tsp)

To serve

- Gem lettuces (3 with leaves separated)
- Crabmeat (200g/8oz)
- Bunch chives (1/2)
- Lemon wedges (optional)

HOW TO COOK:

1 Combine all the ingredients for Marie rose sauce and set aside in a refrigerator.

2 Do this for the ingredients for the tomato salsa as well. (they can be prepared ahead for as long as 24 hours.

3   Arrange prawns, lettuce leaves, and chives into separate bowls. Set all on a table along with a pile of lemon wedges

4   Add some prawns & crab to the lettuce leaves. Spoon over some of the Marie Rose sauce and tomato salsa then scatter over some chives. You may also add a squeeze of lemon if you desire.

GREEK SALAD OMELETTE

TIME: 20 MINUTES
AMOUNT:4 TO 6 SERVINGS

Calories-371kcal
Protein-24g
Fat-28g
Carbs-5g

INGREDIENTS:

- ♦ Eggs (10)
- ♦ Parsley leaves (chopped, a handful)-optional
- ♦ Olive oil (2 tbsp)
- ♦ Red onion (1, cut into wedges)
- ♦ Tomatoes (3, chopped into big chunks)
- ♦ Black olives (a handful, pitted)
- ♦ Feta cheese (100g/4oz, crumbled)

HOW TO COOK:

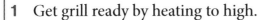

| 1 | Get grill ready by heating to high. |

| 2 | Whisk eggs & fresh parsley in a bowl. Add pepper & salt |

| 3 | Heat oil in a skillet then fry onion until it is browned around its edges (about 4 minutes). Add in olives and tomatoes then leave to cook for2 minutes till the tomatoes start to soften. |

| 4 | Turn the heat down to medium then pour in eggs. Cook for about 3 minutes. Ensure that you stir as you cook.Turn off the heat when egg is halfcooked but runny in some places. |

| 5 | Scatter over feta cheese then place pan under grill for 5 minutes until omelet become puffed and turns golden. |

| 6 | Cut into wedges and serve immediately. |

GOAN MUSSELS

TIME: 30 MINUTES
AMOUNT4 SERVINGS

Calories-291kcal
Protein-14g
Fat-23g
Carbs-9g

INGREDIENTS:

- Fresh mussel (1 kg/2lbs)
- Sunflower oil
- Onion (1, chopped)
- Ginger (thumb sized, grated)
- Garlic (4 cloves, crushed)
- Green chiñlies (2 chopped)
- Ground turmeric (1 tsp)
- Ground Coriander (2 tsp)
- Coriander sprigs and lime wedges (to serve)

HOW TO COOK:

1. Remove beards from mussels and wash in cold water a couple of times until it is clean and clear. Discard broke mussels or those that stay open when tapped

2. Heat oil in a pan or flameproof casserole. Fry onion in the oil till lightly browned. Add garlic, spices, ginger & chilies. Season with pepper & salt.

3. Cook in for 2 to 3 minutes till fragrant & toasted.

4   Pour in the coconut milk and bring to boil. Simmer for some minutes

5   Tip mussel into dish & turn the heat up with the covered for 3 to 4 minutes till the mussels are just opened.

6   Turn down heat and scatter with coriander sprigs. You can serve with lime wedges if desired.

AUBERGINE MELTS

TIME: 30 MINUTES
AMOUNT:4 SERVINGS

Calories-213kcal
Protein-9g
Fat-17g
Carbs-7g

INGREDIENTS:

- Aubergines (2, halved lengthwise)
- Tomatoes (4)
- Olive oil
- Mozzarella (150g/6oz, drained)
- Basil leaves (a handful)

HOW TO MAKE:

1	Get the oven ready by heating to 200C/380F

2	Drizzle oil over aubergines and place in the oven then bake for 24 minutes till softened.

3	Meanwhile, slice mozzarella & tomatoes and place them on top of the aubergines.

4	Return to oven then bake for 5 more minutes to melt cheese.

5	Scatter over basil leaves then serve. Can be served with green salad and couscous.

CEVICHE

TIME:20 MINUTES
AMOUNT:6 SERVINGS

Calories-154kcal
Protein-19g
Fat-6g
Carbs-6g

INGREDIENTS:

- Juice (from 8 limes)
- Lime wedges (to serve)
- Onions (1 red, cut into rings)
- White fish fillets (500g/1 lbs, firm)
- Green olives (a handfull, finely chopped)
- Green chillies (3, finely chopped)
- Tomatoes(2 or 3. de-seeded then chopped)
- Bunch coriander (roughly chopped)
- Olive oil (2 tbsp)
- Caster sugar
- Tortilla chips (for serving)

HOW TO COOK:

1   Mix fish, lime, lime juice and onion inside a bowl. The juice should cover the fish completely. You may add more lime if the quantity you have is not sufficient.

2   Cover bowl with a cling film then place on a fridge for about 1 hr 30 minutes

3   Remove onion and fish from lime juice and discard juice.

4   Add olives, tomatoes, coriander, olive oil and chillies to a bowl containing fish and onions. Mix gently. Add salt to taste

5   Once mixture is ready you can store in a fridge until needed.

6   To serve, scoop ceviche into a serving bowl along with tortilla chips.

STEAMED FISH AND PAK CHOI PARCELS

TIME: 30 MINUTES
AMOUNT: 4 SERVINGS

Calories-124kcal
Protein-22g
Fat-3g
Carbs-2g

INGREDIENTS:

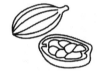

- White fish fillets (4 Plaice)
- 2 pak choi (sliced thickly)
- Spring onion (4, shredded)
- Red chilli (1, sliced thinly)
- Ginger (cut into matchsticks)
- Juice (from one lime)
- Soy sauce (low salt)
- Sesame oil(1 tsp)

HOW TO COOK:

1   Get oven ready by heating to 380F/180C

2   Place ach fish fillet on a foil and top with pak choi, chilli, spring onions and ginger. Pull up the wedges of the foil

3   Mix lime juice and soy sauce along with 1 tbsp of water. Spoon a little of this over each fillet.

4   Enclose the fish in the foil by crimping the top part of the foil. Ensure there is no gap in the foil that will allow steam to escape.

5 Place the parcels on baking pan then bake in the oven for 14 minutes till cooked through. (you may spend less or more time depending on how thick the fish fillets are).

6 Open the parcels and add some sesame oil as drizzle.

7 Serve with rice or as desired.

PRAWN AND CHORIZO

TIME: 35 MINUTES
AMOUNT:2 SERVINGS

Calories-390kcal
Protein-34g
Fat-25g
Carbs-8g

INGREDIENTS:

- ◆ Onion (1/2, chopped)
- ◆ Chorizo (50g/2oz, sliced)
- ◆ Olive oil (2 tsp)
- ◆ Eggs (4, lightly beaten)
- ◆ Milk (1 tbsp)
- ◆ Peeled prawn (85g/3oz)
- ◆ Frozen pea (100g, defrosted)
- ◆ Leafy salad (to serve)

HOW TO COOK:

1	Heat grill on medium setting

2	Fry onion and chorizo over low heat. Cook for 5 minutes to soften onions. Be sure to stir as you cook.

3	Remove the pan from the heat. Remove any excess far left from cooking chorizo. Stir in the eggs and milk then add seasoning.

4	Stir in peas & prawn and cook for 13 minutes on low heat till all parts of the fritata except the top is set.

5	Flash fritata under grill till color turns golden.

6	Can be served with leafy salad as desired.

CHEESE AND ONION PORK CHOPS

TIME: 20 MINUTES
AMOUNT:4 SERVINGS

Calories-379kcal
Protein-36g
Fat-23g
Carbs-8g

INGREDIENTS:

- Pork chops (4)
- Olive oil (2 tsp)
- English mustard (1 tsp)
- Caramelized onions (4 tbsp)
- Cheshire cheese (50g/2oz, grated)
- Thyme (chopped, 1 tsp)

HOW TO COOK:

1	Prepare grill by heating on high settings.

2	Place porks on a grill pan then rub with oil. Add seasoning & place on grill for about 6 minutes ob each side till color turns golden.

3	Spread some mustard over one side of each pork chop. Top this with 1 tbsp of onion for each. Make a mixture of thyme and cheese. Sprinkle this over the chops.

4	Return to grill & cook for some minutes until it is bubbly with a golden color.

MAC & CHEESE WITH ZUCCHINI NOODLES

TIME: 25 MINUTES
AMOUNT:4 SERVINGS

Calories-242kcal
Protein-36g
Fat-20g
Carbs-19g

INGREDIENTS:

- Zucchinis (4 lbs/1.8kg) spiralized with a blade
- Salt
- Mozzarella cheese (lightly packed, 1.5c)
- Grated Parmesan cheese (3/4c)
- Sundried tomatoes (1/2c, with Italian herbs)
- Non-fat Greek yogurt (1/2c)
- Garlic salt (1 tsp)
- Pepper
- Italian seasoning (1 tsp)
- Basil (fresh)

HOW TO MAKE:

1   Boil salted water in a pot. Add zucchini noodles to boiling water. Break very long noddles as you add them to the pot. Cook for 3 minutes.

2   Drain noodles by pouring into a colander. Return pot to heat and turn down to medium low.

3   Shake water from the noodles and further dry off using double layers of a kitchen towel. Squeeze the noodles with the towels to get as much water out as possible. (do not grab the towel directly since the water will be hot and you can burn yourself).

4   Transfer noodles to a layer of paper towel to further squeeze water out. Repeat this with a new layer of towel.

5   Return noodles to the pot. Stir in cheese, a handful at a time. Add more cheese as the previous batch melts.

6   Once you have added all the cheese and it has all melted, add in Greek yogurt and stir until well combined.

7   Stir in the garlic salt, sun dried tomatoes, Italian seasoning and pepper.

8   To be served with fresh basil as garnish if desired.

CHEESY PIZZA CHICKEN

TIME: 50 MINUTES
AMOUNT: 6 SERVINGS

Calories-228kcal
Protein-11g
Fat-6g
Carbs-6g

INGREDIENTS:

♦ Chicken breasts (2, cut into two)

♦ Garlic powder (1 tbsp)

♦ Italian seasoning (1 tsp)

♦ Olive oil(2 tbsp)

♦ Pasta sauce (1 cup)

♦ Sea salt(1 tbsp)

♦ Mozzarella (1 cup)

♦ Parmesan (1/4 cup)

♦ Pepperoni (12)

♦ Cilantro (optional)

HOW TO COOK:

| 1 | Get oven ready by preheating to 190C/375F |

| 2 | Butterfly the chicken breasts then cut into two |

| 3 | Season each piece with herbs and salt |

| 4 | Add oil to a pan and heat then add chicke in batches. Brown for about 3 minutes in the oil on each side. |

5   Add chicken to a baking sheet, top with sauce, herbs and cheese

6   Add pepperonis on the chicken. Place in oven and bake for 24 to 30 minutes till the cheese melts and the chicken is well cooked.

7   Serve with cilantro as toppings.

LOW CARB PALEO MEATLOAF

TIME: 1 HOUR 10 MINS
AMOUNT: 6 SERVINGS

Calories-208kcal
Protein-18g
Fat-12g
Carbs-8g

INGREDIENTS:

For Sauce

- Canned tomato sauce (1/2 cup)
- Tomato paste (1/4c)
- Deglet Noor dates (2 tbsp)
- Water (2 tbsp)
- Garlic powder
- Sea salt (1/2 tsp)
- White Vinegar (1 tbsp)
- Onion Powder (1 tsp)

For Meatloaf

- Ground beef (0.45kg/1lb)
- Egg (1 large)
- Green bell pepper (6 tbsp, diced)
- Sea salt (1/2 tsp)
- Green onion (1/4c, sliced)
- A pinch of black pepper
- Coconut flour (4 tsp)

HOW TO COOK:

1	Get oven ready by preheating to 180C/350F

2	Mix all ingredient for sauce in a pot and bring to boil.

3 Stir frequently as you cook. Turn down the temperature to medium after boiling for 2 minutes & cook for some minutes to thicken the sauce.

4 Transfer sauce to a food processor, blend till the sauce is smooth & the dates are well incorporated.

5 Mix all the ingredients for the meatloaf (except coconut flour) with your hands in a medium bowl. Add in coconut flour then mix till well incorporated.

6 Transfer meatloaf mixture to a pan and press to form an even layer. (do not overpack). Spread sauce over the top then bake for about 50 minutes until meatloaf is no longer pink.

7 Leave for 5 minutes to cool then serve.

DINNER RECIPES

BARLEY CHICKEN AND MUSHROOM RISOTTO

TIME: 1 HOUR
AMOUNT:4 SERVINGS

Calories-546kcal
Protein-42g
Fat-12g
Carbs-61g

INGREDIENTS:

- Olive oil (1 tbsp)
- Shallots (2, finely sliced)
- Butter (1 tbsp)
- Garlic (1 clove, chopped)
- Chicken breasts (3, skinless)
- Pearl barley (300g/10oz)
- White wine (250ml)
- Wild & chestnut mushroom (400g/14oz, chopped)
- Thyme leaf (1 tbsp)
- Parmesan cheese (3 tbsp, grated)
- Chicken stock(1L)
- Chives(snipped)-optional
- Parmesan shavings-optional

HOW TO MAKE:

1   In a large saucepan melt oil and butter. Pour in shallot & garlic with seasoning and saute for about 5 minutes. Add in chicken (cut into chunks) & cook for 2 additional minutes.

2   Add barley to the saucepan & cook for a minutes. Pour in white wine and continue to stir until all the wine is absorbed.

3   Add thyme and mushroom. Pour in 3/4 of the stock. Continue to cook on a low simmering heat for 40 minutes to tenderize barley. Stir as your cook & add more of the e stock if it becomes too dry.

4   Turn down the heat then stir in in grated Parmesan.

5   To be served immediately with the Parmesan shavings and chives if desired.

MEXICAN CHICKEN STEW

TIME:45 MINUTES
AMOUNT: 4 SERVINGS

Calories-203kcal
Protein-35g
Fat-5g
Carbs-6g

INGREDIENTS:

- ◆ Vegetable oil (1tbsp)
- ◆ Garlic (3 cloves, finely chopped)
- ◆ Brown sugar (1/2 tsp)
- ◆ Chipotole paste (1 tsp)
- ◆ Onion (1, finely chopped)
- ◆ Chopped tomatoes (1 400g/14oz can)
- ◆ Red onion (1 small, sliced into rings)
- ◆ Coriander leaves (a few)
- ◆ Rice or Corn tortillas (to serve)

HOW TO COOK:

1 In a medium saucepan, add oil then onions and saute for 4 minutes until onions are softened. Add in garlic then cook for 1 additional minute. Stir in chipotole paste, tomatoes and sugar.

2 Add chicken into this pan & spoon over the sauce. Leave for 18 to 20 minutes to simmer gently. (you can add some water if the sauce gets too dry).

3 Turn down the heat and remove chicken from pan. Shred chicken with forks & return into the sauce. Add red onion and coriander.

4 Remove from t he heat when done & service with rice or corn tortillas.

LOW CARB SPINACH DIP CHICKEN

TIME: 35 MINUTES
AMOUNT:4 SERVINGS

Calories-374kcal
Protein-44g
Fat-15.4g
Carbs-12g

INGREDIENTS:

- Frozen spinach (8oz, 230g)
- Chicken breast (1lb/0.45kg)
- Greek yogurt (1 1/2 cups)
- Neufchatel cheese (8oz/230g, softened)
- Mozzarella cheese (part skim, 1/2c)
- Garlic cloves (2)
- Pepper & salt

HOW TO COOK:

1	Get oven ready by preheating to 360F/180C

2	Follow the instruction on the package to cook frozen spinach. Remove from the heat & leave aside to cool. Once cooled, remove excess moisture from spinach using paper towels.

3	Mix Greek yogurt, Neufchatel and frozen spinach. Add in the garlic then add salt and pepper to season as desired.

4	Place chicken breast on the pan then season with more pepper & salt.

5	Spread the spinach mixture on the chicken evenly then sprinkle with mozzarella cheese.

6	Bake in oven for about 23 to 28 minutes until cooked through.

7	To be served immediately.

SEA BASS WITH FENNEL, LEMON AND SPICES

TIME: 25 MINUTES
AMOUNT:2 SERVINGS

Calories-241kcal
Protein-32g
Fat-10g
Carbs-6g

INGREDIENTS:

- Fennel seed (1 tsp)
- Cumin seed (1 tsp)
- Mustard seed (1 tsp)
- Fennel bulb (1, finely sliced)
- Turmeric (1 tsp)
- Sea bass (1 small, descaled and gutted)
- Lemon (1, finely sliced + wedges)-to serve, optional
- Coriander leaves (a handful) to serve.

HOW TO COOK:

1   Prepare oven by preheating to 220C/400F

2   Combine all the spices. Brush a large square of foil with some oil then scatter over fennel. Sprinkle with 1/3 of the spices, 1/2 the chili and some of the seasoning.

3   Rub the remaining spices and chilli on the fish (both inside and outside). Place fish on top of fennel seeds then stuff with lemon slices.

4   Bring the edges of the foil together & seal well. Place the parcel on a tray and put in oven to cook for 12 to 15 minutes.

5   Unwrap, scatter with coriander leaves then serve with lemon wedges if desired.

LOW-CARB CREAMY SOUTHWEST CHICKEN

TIME: 25 MINUTES
AMOUNT:4 SERVINGS

Calories-191kcal
Protein-15g
Fat-13g
Carbs-3g

INGREDIENTS:

- ♦ Chicken breast (2 medium, bone & skin removed)
- ♦ Onion (minced, 1/4 cup)
- ♦ Olive oil (1 tbsp)
- ♦ Garlic (minced, 2 cloves,)
- ♦ Green chilies (4.5oz/130g)
- ♦ Cheddar cheese (1/4 cup, shredded)
- ♦ Heavycream (1/4 cup)

HOW TO COOK:

1   Pour oil into a large skillet placed over medium heat.

2   Cut chicken breast into bite-size pieces then add salt & pepper to season. Saute in the oil until both sides are browned. Add onions halfway through cooking.

3   Add garlic then cook for 1 additional minute.

4   You may add water to de-glaze the pan if needed.

5   Add cream and green chilies to pan. Leave to simmer till the chicken is done and the sauce has thickened.

6   Top with cheddar cheese and serve when the cheese melts.

LOW CARB TURKEY TETRAZZINI RECIPE

TIME: 40 MINUTES
AMOUNT:8 SERVINGS

Calories-226kcal
Protein-21g
Fat-12g
Carbs-8g

INGREDIENTS:

- Chopped turkey (3 cups)
- Spaghetti squash (6 cups, cooked)
- Mushrooms (8 oz, sliced)
- Oil (2 tsp)
- Soy milk (Unsweetened, 1 1/2 cup)
- Cream (/2 cup)
- Flour or any other thickener (optional)
- Almond meal (1/4 cup)
- Parmesan cheese (grated, 1/4c)- optional
- Dry sherry (1/3 cup)-optional
- Salt and pepper (to taste)

HOW TO COOK:

1 Saute onions in oil and butter for a while. Add in mushroom & cook until almost dry. Season with salt & pepper. Stir as you cook. (you may thicken with flour if desired and bring to simmer for a few minutes). Add sherry if desired as well.

2 Add in turkey then leave for a few minutes to simmer to cook turkey through.

3 Mix with squash or noddles in a casserole pan.

4 Sprinkle some cheese and almond meal as topping. Bake for about 10 minutes in oven till toppings are browned.

COCONUT CURRY CHICKEN RECIPE

TIME: 30 MINUTES
AMOUNT: SERVES 4

INGREDIENTS:

- Coconut oil (1 tbsp)
- Onion (chopped, 1/2 medium)
- Curry paste (2 tbsp)
- Red bell pepper (1 medium, cored, seeded then chopped)
- Salt
- Chicken thighs (0.45kg/1lb, bones & skin removed, then cut in bite-size pieces)
- Coconut milk (3/4 of a 14oz/400g can)
- Green beans (frozen or fresh, 12oz/340g)
- Juice (from 1 lime)

HOW TO COOK:

1 Pour the oil into a large skillet to form a think coating at the base.

2 Add the chopped onions and red bell pepper. Stir and continue to cook until onions becomes soft and translucent.

3 Add Thai spices. Season with salt. And stir continuously as you cook till you begin to smell the spices.

4 Add chopped chicken & cook until the chicken is almost cooked through.

5   Add the unsweetened coconut milk and the fresh or frozen green beans then bring to boil until green beans are al dente.

6   Remove from heat then serve with lime juice.

LOW-CARB BEEF FAJITAS

TIME: 30 MINUTES
AMOUNT:5 FAJITAS

Calories-283kcal
Protein-38g
Fat-12g
Carbs-5g

INGREDIENTS:

- Skirt steak (2 lbs/0.9kg, cut into strips)
- 1 medium onion (sliced)
- 2 large bell peppers (large)
- Soy sauce (1/4c)
- Lime juice (1/4c)
- Chilli powder (1 tsp)
- Oil (2 tbsp)

HOW TO MAKE:

| 1 | Mix soy sauce, chilli powder and lime juice with oil |

| 2 | Cut meat into slices (about 1/2 inch each) cut perpendicular to the grain. |

| 3 | Marinate meat in plastic bag for a few minutes |

| 4 | Cook meat in batches until each piece is browned. Turn down the heat then add in vegetables. Return meat to the skillet when the veggies become soft then heat through until well cooked. |

| 5 | To be served with salsa, cilantro or sour cream if desired. |

GRILLED STEAK SALAD WITH HORSERADISH DRESSING

TIME: 15 MINUTES
AMOUNT: 2 SERVINGS

Calories-305kcal
Protein-30g
Fat-18g
Carbs-6g

INGREDIENTS:

- Skirt steak (9oz/250g)
- Celery seeds (1 tsp, crushed)
- Olive oil (for brushing)
- Celery(6 sticks, thinly sliced)
- Worcestershire sauce (1 tbsp)
- Mixed tomato(plum, red, beefsteak & yellow) 200g/7oz

For Dressing

- Worcestershire sauce (1 tbsp)
- Olive oil (1 tbsp)
- Horseradish sauce (1 tsp)
- Red wine vinegar (1 tsp)
- Tomato puree (1 tsp)

HOW TO COOK:

1 Rub steak on both sides with crushed celery seeds, Worcestershire sauce and some seasoning.

2 Brush the seasoning with olive oil then leave to marinate while you get the salad ready.

3 Mix all the dressing ingredients in a small bowl.Divide tomatoes and celery into 2 plates.

4   Place pan over high heat and add oil. Cook meat for about 3 minutes on each side.

5   Remove from heat then set aside to cool covered with foil about 5 minutes.

6   Slice steaks & place on top of the salads. Pour dressing over steaks.

LOW CARB BACON CHEESEBURGER CASSEROLE

TIME: 1 HOUR
AMOUNT: 6 SERVINGS

Calories-582kcal
Protein-43g
Fat-43g
Carbs-2g

INGREDIENTS:

- Bacon (250g/ 0.5lb)
- Ground beef (0.45kg/1 lb)
- Sweet onion (1/2)
- Garlic (1 clove)
- Cream cheese (3-4 tbsp)
- Ketchup (2 tbsp, reduced sugar)
- Worcestershire sauce (1 tbsp)
- Salt (1 tsp)
- Yellow mustard (1 tbsp)
- Heavy cream (1/4c)
- Eggs (4 large)
- Hot sauce (1 tsp)
- Cheddar cheese (8oz/226g, grated)
- Fresh dill (1 tsp)
- Ground pepper (1 tsp)

HOW TO COOK:

1   Dice the bacon then place in a skillet. Cook over medium heat until crisp. Stir continuously as you cook. Remove bacon from pan and leave aside. Drain the grease from the meat.

2   Add ground beef to pan and cook till browned. Crumble as you cook. Drain off fat.

3   Add onion & garlic to skillet then add beef. Cook for 5 to 7 minutes until onions are translucent.

4   Add mustard, cream cheese, salt, ketchup and Worcestershire sauce to the skillet and continue to cook over low heat. Stir as it cooks until well mixed.

5   Spread beef mixture into an oiled baking dish then top with the cooked bacon.

6   Break eggs into a bowl & whisk with heavy cream to combine. Stir in hot sauce & pepper. Pour this mixture over bacon and beef then top with cheddar cheese.

7   Bake for 30 minutes in the oven until color turns golden at the top. Serve Sprinkled with dill.

CAULIFLOWER FRIED RICE

TIME: 15 MINUTES
AMOUNT:4 SERVINGS

Calories-152kcal
Protein-5.9g
Fat-10g
Carbs-10g

INGREDIENTS:

- Cauliflower (1/2 head)
- Olive oil (2 tbsp)
- Garlic (2 cloves, minced)
- Carrots (2, diced)
- White onion (1/2 cup, chopped)
- Eggs(2)
- Soy sauce (2 tbsp)
- Frozen peas (1/2c)
- Sesame oil (1/2 tsp, toasted)

HOW TO COOK:

1　Cut cauliflower into smaller chunks then throw into a food processor. Blitz a few times to form rice.

2　Add garlic, onion and carrot into a large wok and cook in the olive oil to tenderize (for 5 minutes).

3　Stir cauliflower rice and frozen peas. Cook for about 5 minutes (with the pot covered) to tenderize cauliflower slightly.

4　Make a hold at the center of the mixture that reaches the base of the wok. Crack eggs into the hold formed and cook till eggs are scrambled. Stir till mixture is combined evenly.

5　Stir in soy sauce & sesame oil & serve warm.

LOW CARB TACO SKILLET

TIME: 15 MINUTES
AMOUNT:6 SERVINGS

Calories-301kcal
Protein-23g
Fat-19g
Carbs-11g

INGREDIENTS:

- Ground turkey (1 lb/0.45 kg)
- Riced cauliflower (12oz/340g, frozen)
- Taco seasoning (1/4 cup)
- Diced tomatoes (1/2 cup)
- 1 Avocado (diced)
- Black beans (1/4cup)
- Lettuce (chopped, 1 cup)
- Cheddar cheese (shredded, 1/4 c)
- Onion (2 tbsp, diced)
- Cilantro (minced, 1 tbsp)

HOW TO COOK:

1 Cook & crumble ground turkey inside a skillet placed over medium high heat.

2 Stir in the Cauliflower rice. Add taco seasoning & 1/4 cup of water. Cook while stirring continuously until cauliflower is heated through

3 Turn off the heat then add lettuce, tomatoes, onions, black beans & cheese to top.

4 Can be served garnished with cilantro.

SNACK RECIPES

NUTTY CHICKEN SATAY STRIPS

TIME: 20 MINUTES
AMOUNT: 2 SERVINGS

Calories-276kcal
Protein-41g
Fat-10g
Carbs-3g

INGREDIENTS:

- Peanut butter (oil & sugar-free, 2 tbsp)
- Garlic (1 clove, grated)
- Curry powder (1 tsp)
- Soy sauce
- Lime juice (2 tsp)
- Chicken (2, skinless)
- Breast fillets (cut into strips)
- Cucumber (cut into fingers)
- Sweet chilli sauce

HOW TO COOK:

5	Get oven ready by preheating to 200C/360F

6	Mix chunky peanut butter with grated garlic clove. Add curry powder and a few shakes of the soy sauce along with 2 tsp of lime juice into a large bowl. You may add little boiling water if the nut butter seems to be too thick.

7	Add strips of chicken breast fillet and mix well. Arrange on baking sheets but be sure to leave enough space between them.

8	Bake in oven for about 10 minutes till well cooked.

9	To be served warm with cucumber the sweet chilli sauce.

AUBERGINE & CHICKPEA BITES

TIME: 1 HR 20 MINUTES
AMOUNT:20 BITES

Calories-66kcal
Protein-2g
Fat-3g
Carbs-5g

INGREDIENTS:

- Aubergines (3, large)-halved with the cut side scored
- Spray oil
- Garlic (2 fat cloves, peeled)
- Coriander (2 tsp)
- Chickpeas (400g can, drained)
- Flour (2 tbsp)
- Cumin seeds (2 tsp)
- Lemon wedges (1/2 lemon)
- Polenta (3 tbsp)
- Lemon zest (from 1/2 lemon)

For dip

- Coconut yogurt (150g/5oz)
- Harissa (1 tbsp)

HOW TO COOK

1   Get oven ready by heating to 200C/380F

2   Spray the aubergine halves with oil then cut side up into a large roasting tin along with the garlic. Add in cumin seeds and coriander then season as desired. Roast in oven for 40 minutes to tenderize aubergine. Place aside to cool.

3 Scoop aubergine flesh into bowl and discard the skin. With a spatula, scrape the garlic and spices into a bowl. Add in chickpeas, flour, lemon juice and zest. Mash all together until well mixed then taste to check seasoning.

4 Form mixture into balls (about 20 balls in all) and place them on baking tray. Put the tray in the fridge for about 30 minutes.

5 Swirl harrisa through the yogurt then set aside.

6 Roll the balls in a bowl of polenta to coat then return them to the baking tray and spray with some oil.

7 Roast in oven for 20 minutes till crisp. You can serve with lemon wedges and harissa yogurt.

MATCHA CASHEW COCONUT ENERGY BALLS

TIME: 10 MINUTES
AMOUNT:12 SERVINGS

Calories-66kcal
Protein-2g
Fat-3g
Carbs-5g

INGREDIENTS:

- Raw cashews (1 cup, soaked 6 -8 hours prior)
- Date paste (3/4 cup, softened in warm water for a while)
- Coconut oil (3 tbsp)
- Unsweetened coconut (1 cup, shredded)
- Matcha tea powder (1 tbsp)

HOW TO COOK:

| 1 | Pour all ingredients into a high powered blender or food processor then blend until well mixed |

| 2 | Roll into tablespoon sized balls and coat with shredded coconut |

| 3 | Leave aside for an hour in the refrigerator to cool before serving. |

SALT & VINEGAR ZUCCHINI CHIPS

TIME: 12 HOURS 10 MINS
AMOUNT:6-SERVINGS

Calories-40kcal
Protein-0.7g
Fat-3.6g
Carbs-2.9g

INGREDIENTS:

- Thinly sliced zucchini (4 cups)
- Avocado oil or extra virgin olive oil (2 tbsp)
- Coarse sea salt (2 tsp)
- White balsamic vinegar (2 tbsp)

HOW TO COOK:

| 1 | Slice zucchini as thin as possible (you can use a mandolin for this). |

| 2 | In a small bowl, add oil and vinegar and whisk to mix. |

| 3 | In a large bowl, place zucchini slices then toss with the oil-vinegar mixture |

| 4 | Add zucchini to a dehydrator in even layers then sprinkle with some coarse sea salt. Drying time on dehydrator may vary from 8 to 14 hours depending on how thin zucchini slices are and the dehydrator being used. |

| 5 | Line cookie sheet with parchment sheet, lay zucchini on sheets evenly & bake in the oven for 3 hour. Rotate half-way though cooking |

| 6 | It can be stored in a closed airtight container. |

NO BAKE PROTEIN BAR RECIPE

TIME: 5 MINUTES
AMOUNT: 12 BARS

INGREDIENTS:

- Gluten free oats (2.5cups)
- Protein powder (1 or 2 scoops)
- Almondbutter (1c)
- Chocolate chip (1/2 cup, optional)
- Pure maple syrup (1/2c)

HOW TO COOK:

1	Prepare 8 x 8-inch pan by lining it with a parchment sheet & set aside
2	In a large bowl, mix protein powder & rolled oats & mix thoroughly.
3	Heat up almond butter and syrup on a microwave safe bowl until well warmed and whisk.
4	Pour wet mixture into the dry mixture and mix thoroughly until well combined. Add a little milk to thin out batter if it is too crumbly.
5	Transfer protein bar batter into the pan and press in place firmly. Refrigerate till firm then slice into bars.
6	Serve drizzled with optional chocolate if desired.

LOW CARB GOLD FISH CRACKERS

TIME: 35
AMOUNT:60 CRACKERS

Calories-52kcal
Protein-1g
Fat-4g
Carbs-1g

INGREDIENTS:

♦ Celtic sea salt (1/8 tsp)

♦ Blanched almond flour (1¼ cup)

♦ Baking soda (1/8 tsp)

♦ Olive oil (1tbsp)

♦ Cheddar cheese (freshly grated, 1 cup)

♦ 1 large Egg

HOW TO COOK:

| 1 | Add baking soda, almond flour & cheese into a blender/food processor and blitz. |

| 2 | Add in eggs and oil then pulse until well mixed |

| 3 | Divide dough formed into two portions |

| 4 | Place one portion of dough in-between 2 parchment sheet and roll until it is about ¼-inch thick. |

| 5 | Remove the parchment sheet's top layer. |

| 6 | Cut out little gold fish shapes using a goldfish cookie cutter |

7   Roll the leftover portion of dough and refrigerate. Cut into goldfish shape as well.

8   Bake dough for about 15 minutes in the oven.

9   Remove from the oven when done, leave to cool for a while then serve.

SIMPLE GRAIN-FREE GRANOLA

TIME: 30 MINUTES
AMOUNT: 20 SERVINGS

Calories-205kcal
Protein-4.3g
Fat-18g
Carbs-9g

INGREDIENTS:

- Coconut flakes (1/2 cup, unsweetened)
- Raw almonds (2 cups, slivered)
- Raw pecans (1 1/4c)
- Chia seeds (3 tbsp)
- Raw walnuts (1 cup)
- Flaxseed meal (1 tbsp)
- Coconut or muscavado or cane sugar (2 tbsp)
- Ground cinnamon (1 1/2 tsp)
- Sea salt (1/4 tsp)
- Olive or coconut oil (3 tbsp_
- Maple syrup (1/3 cup)
- Dried blueberries (1/2 cup, optional)
- Unsalted sunflower seeds (roasted, 1/2 cup) optional

HOW TO COOK:

| 1 | Heat oven to 325F/162C. position a rack at the center of the oven |

| 2 | In a large bowl, mix coconut, chia seeds, flax seeds, cinnaomon, salt and coconut sugar. |

| 3 | Warm oil in a saucepan over low heat. Add maple syrup & pour over dry ingredient then combine well. |

4   Spread mixture formed evenly on a large baking sheets (you may need 2 sheets). Place in preheated oven and leave to bake for 18 to 20 minutes before removing. Add in dried blueberries and roasted sunflower seeds if you are using then stir.

5   Return to oven & turn up the heat to 340F/171C for 6 -8minutes until color turns a deep golden brown. (the coconut oil will help the granola to crisp nicely, however, be sure to watch it so it doesn't brown too much).

6   Remove Granola from the oven & leave to cool for a while. Serve immediately or store in an airtight container (can be stored for a few weeks).

SOFT PRETZELS (GLUTEN-FREE)

TIME:1 HOUR 40 MINS
AMOUNT: 8 PRETZELS

Calories-200kcal
Protein-15g
Fat-7g
Carbs-13g

INGREDIENTS:

- Psyllium Husk Powder (3 tbsp)
- Active dry yeast (1 tbsp)
- Applesauce (1/2 cup, unsweetened)
- Almond milk (1 cup, unsweetned vanilla flavor)
- Organic soy four (1.5c)
- Baking powder (2 tsp)
- Salt (1/4 tsp)
- Coconut flour (1 1/4c)
- Water (1 tsp)
- Egg yolk (from 1 large egg)
- Baking soda (1/2 tsp)
- Egg whites (from5 eggs)
- Flaked sea salt (2 tsp)

HOW TO COOK:

1 Mix yeast and psyllium in a small bowl. Also mix almond milk, egg whites, butter favor and apple sauce using a stand mixer on medium speed. Add the psyllium and yeast mixture as you mix until smooth. (the mixture will have a thick gravy look)

2 Mix soy flour, baking powder, baking soda & salt in a bowl. Add this to the mixture in the stand mixer then mix again this time on low speed. (the dough formed will be thick, dense & slightly sticky)

3 Shape dough into a ball and place in a bowl (cover bowl with a plastic wrap. Leave for about an hour in warm place.

4 Preheat oven to 350F/160C and prepare two cookie sheets

5 Divide the dough into equal portions (you should have about 8). Carefully roll dough to form long logs (logs may break, just stick it back together) then shape into pretzels.

6 Transfer pretzels into prepared pans

7 Whisk egg yolk in a small bowl & add water. Brush the pretzels with the egg yolk mixture and sprinkle with salt.

8 Bake in oven until color turns golden brown (about 25 minutes).

9 Leave to cool slightly before serving.

DOUBLE PEANUT BUTTER PROTEIN BALLS

TIME: 10 MINUTES
AMOUNT: 2 SERVINGS

Calories-119kcal
Protein-4g
Fat-7g
Carbs-11g

INGREDIENTS:

- Peanut butter (1 cup, sugar-free)
- Powdered peanut butter (2T)
- Honey (1/4 cup)
- Old fashioned rolled oats (1 1/2 cups)
- Vanilla extract (2 tsp)
- Shredded coconut (1/2 cup) unsweetened
- Mini chocolate chips (1/3c)
- Sea salt

HOW TO COOK:

1 Mix the natural peanut butter and the powdered one with vanilla extract and raw honey inside a medium bowl.

2 Add rolled oats, sea salt, mini chocolate chips & unsweetened coconut and mix thoroughly

3 Form mixture into balls (about 1 inch each) by gently rolling one 1tbsp of the mixture and rolling it in between your palms (you can form into any desired shape). add a little water (one tsp at a time) if the mixture seems to dry).

4 Can be stored in an airtight container and kept for up to a week on the refrigerator.

BASIL AND OLIVE EGGS

TIME: 8 MINUTES
AMOUNT:2 TO 3 SERVINGS

Calories-137kcal
Protein-10g
Fat-11g
Carbs-0.3g

INGREDIENTS:

- Eggs (3)
- Basil (small pack, 1/2)
- Kalamata olives (6, pitted)
- Rapeseed oil (1 tbsp)
- Cidar vinegar (1 tsp)

HOW TO COOK:

| 1 | Boil eggs for 6 to 8 minutes then put in cold water to cool. Peel and cut egg in halve and scoop out yolk. Set egg white aside. Do this for all 6 eggs |

| 2 | Put olives, basil, a grinding of pepper and vinegar into a small bowl. |

| 3 | Blitz using a hand blender. Add egg yolk and mash up together. |

| 4 | Spoon mixture into the egg whites and keep in a fridge. |

SMOOTHIES RECIPES

LOW CARB STRAWBERRY-CHIA SEED SMOOTHIE

TIME: 10 MINUTES
AMOUNT:1 SMOOTHIE

Calories-228kcal
Protein-8g
Fat-19g
Carbs-10g

INGREDIENTS:

- Organic strawberries (3)
- Spinach or kale (1/2 cup, frozen)
- Chia seeds (1 tsp)
- Almond butter (2 tbsp)
- Any Granular sweetener (1 tbsp)
- Cup of water or almond milk

HOW TO MAKE:

| 1 | Pour all your ingredients into a blender cup. |

| 2 | Turn on the blender to blend until smooth. |

| 3 | Serve and enjoy |

LOW-CARB GREEN SMOOTHIE

TIME:5 MINUTES
AMOUNT: 2 SERVINGS

Calories-170kcal
Protein-6g
Fat-14gg
Carbs-7g

INGREDIENTS:

- Spinach (1 cup)
- Coconut milk (1.5c, unsweetened)
- Avocado (1, medium, peeled & pitted)
- 1 scoop Sugar-free vanilla protein powder
- Peanut butter powder (1 tbsp)
- Freshly squeezed lemon (1 tbsp)

HOW TO COOK:

| 1 | Pour all your ingredients into the blender |

| 2 | Puree for 30 seconds. |

| 3 | Taste to see if the flavor needs adjustment |

| 4 | Serve immediately. |

CHOCOLATE PEANUT BUTTER SMOOTHIE

TIME: 10 MINUTES
AMOUNT: 3 SERVINGS

Calories-436kcal
Protein-9g
Fat-41g
Carbs-10g

INGREDIENTS:

- Peanut butter (1/4 cup)
- Heavy creamor coconut cream (1 cup)
- Unsweetened almond milk (1 1/2 cup)
- Cocoa powder(3 tbsp)
- Powdered ertythritol (6 tbsp)
- Sea salt

HOW TO COOK:

| 1 | Pour all your ingredients into a blender and mix |

| 2 | Puree for some seconds. Check smoothness and puree some more if required. |

| 3 | Taste and adjust sweetener if required. |

| 4 | Serve |

LOW CARB BLUEBERRY SMOOTHIE

TIME: 10 MINUTES
AMOUNT:1 SERVING

Calories-216kcal
Protein-24g
Fat-10g
Carbs-7g

INGREDIENTS:

- Coconut milk (1cup)
- Vanilla extract (1tsp)
- Coconut oil or MCT oil (1 tsp)
- Blueberries (1/4 cup)
- Protein powder (30g/1oz optional)

HOW TO COOK:

1	Put all the ingredients into a blender

2	Puree until smooth

3	Serve immediately or chilled

LOW CARB SMOOTHIE WITH ALMOND MILK

TIME: 10 MINUTES
AMOUNT:1 SERVING

Calories-332kcal
Protein-10g
Fat-28g
Carbs-13g

INGREDIENTS:

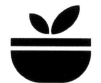

- Almond milk (1 cup)
- Crushed ice (1)
- Avocado (1/4 cup)
- Monkfruit (3tbsp)
- Natural peanut butter (2 tbsp)
- Unsweetened cocoa powder (1 tbsp)

HOW TO COOK:

1	Put all your ingredients into the blender.

2	Turn blender on and blend until smooth

3	Serve.

LOW CARB TASTIEST DESSERTS

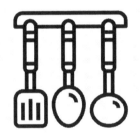

PEANUT BUTTER BARS

TIME:10 MINUTES
AMOUNT: 8 SERVINGS

Calories-246kcal
Protein-7g
Fat-23g
Carbs-7g

INGREDIENTS:

For Bars

- Almondflour (3/4c)
- Butter (2 oz/56g)
- Vanilla extract
- Swerve (1/4 cup)
- Creamy peanut butter (1/2 cup)

For topping

- Chocolate chips(sugar-free, 1/2c)

HOW TO COOK:

| 1 | Mix all ingredients for the bar then spread into on a pan. |

| 2 | Melt chocolate chips in a microwave safe dish for about 30 seconds then stir. |

| 3 | Spread the toppings on the bars. |

| 4 | Can be refrigerated for as long as required for the bar to thicken up. . |

CHOCOLATE CHIPS COOKIE FAT BOMBS

TIME: 45 MINUTES
AMOUNT:30 FAT BOMBS

Calories-137kcal
Protein-2g
Fat-11g
Carbs-10g

INGREDIENTS:

- butter (1/2 cup, softened)
- Swerve (1/3 cup)
- Pure vanilla (1 tsp)
- Almond flour (2 cups)
- Dark chocolate (9oz/255g)
- Kosher salt (1/2 tsp)
- Chocolate chips (8 oz/226g, sugar free)

HOW TO COOK:

1   Beat butter until fluffy and light in a bowl using a hand mixer. Add in sugar, vanilla and salt and mix until well combined.

2   To this, add almond flour one small bit at a time until the dough formed is the right consistency. Add dark chocolate chips & mix.. Leave for 10-15 minutes in the freezer with the bowl covered with plastic wrap.

3   Remove dough from refrigerator and form balls about 1-inch in size using a cookie scoop or spoon. Place balls on baking pan lined with parchment sheet.

4   Melt chocolate chops in a microwave-safe dish fr about 30 seconds. Stir until smooth and completely melted.

5   Dip each fat bomb in the melted chocolate and return to the baking sheet. Leave in the freezer for about 5 minutes to harden.

LOW CARB PEANUT BUTTER MOUSSE

TIME: 5 MINUTES
AMOUNT:4 SERVINGS

Calories-301kcal
Protein-6g
Fat-26g
Carbs-6g

INGREDIENTS:

- Heavy cream (1/2 cup)
- Cream cheese (4 oz/110g)
- Peanut butter (1/4 cup, sugar-free)
- Swerve (1/4 cup)
- Vanilla extract (1/2 tsp)

HOW TO COOK:

1   Whip heavy cream in a bowl until stiff peaks form and set aside.

2   Beat cream cheese & peanut butter together in a bowl until creamy and smooth. Add vanilla, sweetener and a little salt if the peanut butter is unsalted. Beat mixture thoroughly until smooth. (you may add about 2 tbsp of heavy cream if the mixture is thicker than you desire)

3   Gently fold in heavy cream into cream cheese and peanut butter mixture until there is no streaks arc left. Scoop or pipe into dessert glasses to serve.

4   Drizzle with low carb chocolate sauce if desired.

LEMON BARS

TIME: 1 HOUR
AMOUNT:8 SERVINGS

Calories-271kcal
Protein-8g
Fat-26g
Carbs-4g

INGREDIENTS:

♦ Butter (melted, 1/ 2 cup)

♦ Almond flour (1 3/4c)

♦ Powdered erythritol (1 cup, divided)

♦ Lemon (3, medium)

♦ Eggs (3, large)

HOW TO COOK:

1 Mix butter, almond flour (1 cup), erythritol (1/4 cup) and some salt.

2 Press the mixture into a lined baking dish. Place dish in oven & bake for 20 minutes.

3 Remove from oven and set aside to cool.

4 To prepare filling, zest one lemon and juice all three. Mix with eggs, remaining erythritol & almond flour in a bowl then season with a pinch of salt.

5 Pour filling onto to the prepared crust then bake for 20-25 minutes.

6 To be served with a sprinkle of erythritol and lemon slices.

WENDY'S CHOCOLATE FROSTY

TIME: 10 MINUTES
AMOUNT:4 SERVINGS

Calories-241kcal
Protein-3g
Fat-25g
Carbs-3g

INGREDIENTS:

- Heavy cream (1c)
- Cocoa powder (2 tbsp, Unsweetened)
- Vanilla extract (1 tsp)
- Almond butter (1 tablespoon)

HOW TO MAKE:

| 1 | Combine all ingredients and beat until stiff peaks begin to form] |

| 2 | Place mixture in a freezer and leave for about 30 to 60 minutes till barely frozen |

| 3 | Cut on one corner and serve into small cups. |

CINNAMON ROLL FLATBREAD

TIME: 25 MINUTES
AMOUNT: 8 SERVINGS

Calories-171kcal
Protein-7g
Fat-24g
Carbs-5g

INGREDIENTS:

For Dough

- Coconut flour (1/3c)
- Baking powder (1/2 tsp)
- Swerve(2 tbsp)
- Salt (1/8 tsp)
- Mozzarella cheese (shredded, 1.5cups)
- Cream cheese (1 tbsp)
- Cinnamon (1/2 tsp)
- Heavy whipping cream (2 tbsp)
- Eggs (2, large, slightly beaten)

For Topping:

- Butter (melted, 3 tbsp)
- Swerve (3 tbsp, brown)
- Vanilla extract (1/8 tsp)
- Swerve confectioners (2.5 tbsp)
- Cinnamon (1/2 tsp)

HOW TO COOK:

1 To prepare dough, prepare baking sheet and heat oven to 425F/200C

2 Mix coconut flour, swerve, baking powder and cinnamon. Add a little salt and set aside for some time.

3   Mix cream cheese & mozzarella in a microwave-safe bowl. Place in a microwave on high heat for about 45 seconds to melt. Remove mixture, stir and spread then return to the microwave again for 45 seconds. Mix until fully combined.

4   Mix eggs, whipping cream and the flour mixture in a large bowl. Add the cheese mixture then knead with your hand to form a dough. Place the dough on baking sheet and roll out to form a rectangle about 1/3-inches thick. Bake in oven for about 6 minutes. Remove and set aside.

5   To prepare topping, mix ingredients thoroughly then brush the top of bread with it. Return bread to oven and leave for 2 minutes. Remove from oven & leave to cool for about 15 minutes.

6   Cut and serve.

PEANUT BUTTER BALLS

TIME: 20 MINUTES
AMOUNT: 18 SERVINGS

Calories-194kcal
Protein-7g
Fat-17g
Carbs-7g

INGREDIENTS:

- Finely chopped peanuts (1 cup, salted)
- Peanut butter (1 cup)
- Powdered sweetener (1 cup)
- Chocolate chips (8oz/225g)

HOW TO COOK:

1	Mix chopped peanuts, peanut butter with sweetener to form a dough

2	Scoop dough and form into balls (you should have 18 in total). Place balls on lined baking sheet and put into a refrigerator put in a refrigerator until cold

3	Melt chocolate chops in a microwave or on a double boiler. Stir every 30 seconds until it is mostly melted.

4	Dip peanut butter balls into chocolate then return to the wax paper. Return balls to the refrigerator and cool until the chocolate has set.

BUTTERFINGER BARS

TIME: 1 HOUR 30 MINS
AMOUNT:10 SERVINGS

Calories-241kcal
Protein-2g
Fat-12g
Carbs-3g

INGREDIENTS:

- Heavy cream (2 tbsp)
- Coconut oil (4 tbsp)
- Chocolate chips (sugar-free, 1/2 cup)
- Caramel extract (2 tsp)
- Golden erythritol (2/3 cup)
- Pink Himalyan salt (a dash)
- Unsaltedbutter (melted, 1/4 cup)
- Cream cheese (soft, 2 tbsp)
- Peanut butter(organic, 1/4 cup)
- Powdered erythritol (3 tbsp)

HOW TO COOK:

1 Get oven ready by heating to 350F/170C

2 Mix golden erythritol, coconut oil and caramel extract in a small bowl. Spread mixture on a baking pan lined with baking sheet. Bake in oven for 8 to 10 minutes. Remove from oven when melted and bubbly. (do not burn as erythritol can easily cause fire & smoke)

3 Place in freezer and leave to cool.

4 While cooking, mix cream cheese, powdered erythritol and butter with a stand mixer on low speed. Mix until smooth. Add coconut oil, peanut butter & salt then mix.

5   Transfer mixture into a bowl. Remove tray from freezer when cool.

6   Crumble into quarter-sized pieces and fold the crunchy bits into peanut butter mixture gently.

7   Spread mixture onto a baking dish lined with parchment sheet evenly.

8   Place chocolate chips & heavy cream into a small bowl and melt in the microwave.

9   Stir mixture until smooth then pour oven peanut butter-crunch mixture. Smooth out on top until completely covered. Place in a fridge. Remove after 1 hour and serve.

HOSTESS CUPCAKES

TIME: 40 MINUTES
AMOUNT:6 CUPCAKES

Calories-285kcal
Protein-5g
Fat-27g
Carbs-7g

INGREDIENTS:

For Cupcakes

- Almond flour (48g/2oz)
- Golden flaxseed meal (18g/0.7oz)
- Baking powder (1 tsp)
- Xanthan gum (1/4 tsp)
- Coconut flour (8g/0.25oz)
- Heavy cream (2 tsp)
- Grass-fed buttter (56g/2oz, unsalted)
- Kosher salt (1/4 tsp)
- Xylitol or erythritol (1/2 cup)F
- Eggs (2)

For Vanilla Filling

- Butter (56g, unsalted)
- Powdered Erythritol (2 to 4 tbsp)
- Kosher salt
- Vanilla extract(1 tsp)
- Heavy cream (as desired)

For Glaze

- Heavy cream (a desired)
- Chocolate bar (60g/2oz)
- Butter (2 tsp, unsalted)

HOW TO COOK:

1   Prepare oven and line or grease a muffin pan and set aside.

2   Mix coconut flour, xanthan hum, almond flour & baking powder in a bowl until well mixed. Set aside.

3   Add heavy cream, butter and cocoa powder into a microwave-safe bowl. Place in a microwave for 30 seconds to melt. Remove from microwave and leave to cool.

4   Add in sweetener and egg (add in 1 at a time & whisk after putting in each one until completely mixed). you should have a smooth and thick mixture with the sweetener fully dissolved. Add the flour mixture earlier set aside and whisk continously until well blended.

5   Divide the batter formed into the prepared muffin pan. Place muffin pan in the oven and bake for 15 to 18 minutes. Remove from oven & leave aside to cool in the muffin pan.

6   To prepare vanilla filling, add sweetener, butter & salt into a medium bowl. Mix for about 7 minutes using an electric mixer until fluffy and light. Mix vanilla extract (you may add more heavy cream if you desire a lighter filling).

7   To prepare chocolate glaze, heat cream till it starts to bubble. To this, add chocolate and remove from heat. Stir until fully melted then add butter.

8   To serve, cut a hole at the top of each cupcake using a knife or cutter. Spoon or pipe some vanilla buttercream into each cupcake. Closeup the cupcake with the cutout then glaze over in chocolate. You are pipe a swirly squiggle at the top as well.

SEX IN A PAN DESSERT RECIPE

TIME: 45 MINUTES
AMOUNT:16 SERVINGS

Calories-344kcal
Protein-4g
Fat-34g
Carbs-5g

INGREDIENTS:

For Pecan Crust

- Blanched almond flour (1 1/2 cup)
- Pecan meal (1/2 cup)
- Butter (1/3 cup, measured solid)
- Powdered erythritol (2tbsp)

For cream cheese layer

- Heavy cream (1/4 cup)
- Vanilla extract (1/2 tsp)
- Softened cream cheese (150g/8oz)
- Powdered erythritol (1/4cup)

For Chocolate Layer

- Cocoa powder (1/3 cup)
- Heavy cream (1.5c)
- Powdered Erythritol (1/3 cup)
- Vanilla extract (1/2 tsp)

For Whipped Cream Layer

- Heavy cream (1 1/2 cup)
- Powdered erythritol (2 tbsp)
- Vanilla extract (1/2 tsp)
- Dark chocolate (1 oz/28g, sugar free) shaved

HOW TO MAKE:

1   To prepare crust, preheat oven to 350F/160C. line baking dish with a parchment sheet.

2   Mix almond flour, powdered erythritol and pecan meal in a large bowl. Stir in the melted butter until you have a crumbly dough. Press dough evenly onto the lined baking dish. Place in oven and bake for 13 to 14 minutes till it turns a golden color and firm. Leave to cool.

3   To prepare cream cheese layer, while the crust is baking, beat cream, powdered erythritol and vanilla extract together until it forms stiff peaks (use a hand mixer)/ gradually and in softened cream cheese and beat until well mixed. Spread the cream cheese evenly on the crust once it has cooled.

4   While crust is cooling, prepare the chocolate layer by beating heavy cream, vanilla and sweetener until it forms stiff peaks. Add in cocoa powder & beat gradually. Spread chocolate over the layer of cream cheese.

5   To make whipped cream layer beat cream, powdered erythritol and vanilla extract until stiff peaks form. Spread this over the chocolate layer then sprinkle some chocolate shavings on top.

6   Can be refrigerated for 1 hour or for as long as required before serving.

DISCLAIMER

This book contains opinions and ideas of the author and is meant to teach the reader informative and helpful knowledge while due care should be taken by the user in the application of the information provided. The instructions and strategies are possibly not right for every reader and there is no guarantee that they work for everyone. Using this book and implementing the information/recipes therein contained is explicitly your own responsibility and risk. This work with all its contents, does not guarantee correctness, completion, quality or correctness of the provided information. Misinformation or misprints cannot be completely eliminated.

Design: NataliaDesign

Coverpicture: Kiian Oksana // shutterstock.com

Printed by Amazon Italia Logistica S.r.l.
Torrazza Piemonte (TO), Italy

13323303R00064